Dedicated to my best friends Rebecca, Sue, Gwyn, Tammy, and Pilly

Lies My Doctor Told Me: Osteoporosis

Dear Health Conscious Friends,

It's so hard nowadays to get good health information, even at your doctor's office. It's not the doctor's fault, really. Doctors are busy folks, which doesn't leave them time to research and learn after leaving medical school, where they may not have learned accurate or complete information about many topics. What is accepted to be true by the mainstream now, is often just plain wrong. My information is based on real scientific studies showing results counter to the current accepted "facts" - so many of which are just fallacies.

How do doctors stay current with the latest clinical studies, anyway? Currently practicing doctors are getting educational materials from Big Pharma drug reps, who keep their products in the doctors' awareness as much as possible. Is it any wonder that those studies are the ones that were financed by the companies that make the drugs? Do you think that those companies publish any studies that don't conclude good results from their products? Do you really think that YOUR doctor has the time to check to see whether or not those are the only studies that show positive results? Or to search to see if there are other methods to get even better results with fewer side effects?

For that reason, I am publishing this new book with all of the secrets that I know can help so many who need answers for many health problems right now. My prayer is that this series of books will enlighten you to find the solutions to stay healthy now and forever.

Blessings with Love,
Harmony

About the Author

In her newest book, *Lies My Doctor Told Me: Osteoporosis*, Harmony Clearwater Grace reveals the lies that mainstream medicine is telling you about how to regain or maintain strong bones. More importantly, she reveals the little-known methods she has discovered that really do work to give you strong and healthy bones at any age, unlike the dangerous and ineffective drugs and other techniques that your doctor will likely tell you that you need in order to have optimum bone health and lower your risk of fractures.

Harmony is a health researcher and author dedicated to finding and spreading the truth about important health concerns. Harmony is also the author of the bestselling books *HCG Diet Made Simple* and *The HCG Diet Book of Secrets*.

An Important Note from Harmony

If I look younger than you, it's probably because I'm taking care of my bones in a different way. And for the same reason, my arteries are probably less clogged than yours.

Little known fact: People who have stronger bones also have smoother skin.

If you won't do this for your bones, do it for your looks. That's right, bone health and skin health are in lockstep because they both need optimal collagen production.

Skin needs it to be firm and supple.

Bones need it to be strong and flexible.

With the information in this book, you can stay younger on the inside (stronger bones) AND younger on the outside (less wrinkled).

In fact, at The Endocrine Society's 93rd Annual Meeting in Boston, results of a study were presented suggesting that severity of facial wrinkles could predict bone density in early menopause.

http://www.eurekalert.org/pub_releases/2011-06/tes-sof060311.php

Research links for collagen, bone, and skin correlations:
http://www.ncbi.nlm.nih.gov/pubmed/24363926
http://www.ncbi.nlm.nih.gov/pmc/articles/PMC3375270/
http://www.ncbi.nlm.nih.gov/pubmed/19330423
http://www.ncbi.nlm.nih.gov/pubmed/22527725
http://www.ncbi.nlm.nih.gov/pubmed/12110404
http://www.ncbi.nlm.nih.gov/pubmed/11071580
http://www.ncbi.nlm.nih.gov/pubmed/25976422
http://www.ncbi.nlm.nih.gov/pubmed/25997875
http://www.ncbi.nlm.nih.gov/pubmed/23949208

Table of Contents

Acknowledgements

Whenever possible, I cite references to support my opinions, usually from clinical studies or sometimes from the internet. When I cite references that can be accessed from the internet, I may include a shortened URL using TinyURLs throughout this book for your convenience in using the URL links with minimum keystrokes. These URL references are not necessary for full understanding of my reasoning, but provide the actual research links that I used, in case you would like to read further background. As time goes on, the websites for those URLs may be changed or deleted altogether, as the internet is not a static reference, nor under my direct control in terms of how it changes. If you find that any URL link in this book no longer works, I apologize in advance, for, again, these are conditions beyond my control.

If you have any questions or concerns about the data in this book, I am always available through email to offer whatever help and support that I can at:

customer_support@hcgdietmadesimple.com

I am also very interested in hearing your story and how this information has helped you. Please be aware, however, that I am not a medical professional and that I cannot answer medical questions.

We only recommend products that we've either personally checked out ourselves or that come from people we know and trust. For doing so, we may receive compensation. Results are unique. Your results may vary.

Lies My Doctor Told Me: Osteoporosis: How the Latest Medical Research on Bone Drugs and Calcium Could Save Your Bones, Your Heart, and Your Life

You just got your bone density test back.

Your doctor wants you to take Actonel, Fosamax, Boniva, or Prolia.

You don't understand why those calcium chews didn't work for you.

You don't know why this is happening.

You did what your doctor told you to do.

You don't know what you did wrong.

There's a better way.

This is your answer.

In her new book – based on proven facts and over 200 clinical studies – Harmony reveals the special strategies for keeping your bones as strong and healthy as possible. Would a powerful bone-building supplement used by thousands in Japan get your attention? You can start using this radically different unconventional approach TODAY to strengthen your bones. Worried that your bones are getting thin and brittle? Get the bone blueprint for strong flexibility. Bend, don't break!.

Don't waste time and money spending months searching unreliable sources with contradicting data. Let Harmony sort through the fluff and confusion for you, put all the pieces together to figure out what really works, and hand you exactly what you need to know.

She makes it even easier by giving you the names and brands and even links to the exact products needed, so that you don't have to guess or search on your own for them.

You'll learn:

- Why all that calcium you took didn't work
- The most common mistake that most women are making when it comes to bone health – that also makes them more wrinkled
- Which bone-strengthening strategy unknown to the vast majority of doctors works better in peer-reviewed medical research
- Why taking your doctor's advice could disfigure you
- The 11 critical nutrients that can make (or break) your bones
- Why calcium and medication isn't your best answer and the 3 simple things to do instead
- How the medication doctors prescribe can make your bones MORE likely to break over time
- The 15 biggest mistakes you are probably making right now that are damaging your bones
- How what you are doing to try to keep healthy strong bones could actually be causing other diseases in your body
- Why your doctor probably doesn't know about this research
- Secrets of the best cutting-edge medical researchers that you need to know to prevent bone loss and fractures
- Why taking extra calcium without THIS can give you heart disease
- How to reduce your fracture risk by at least 60% with a statistical 95% confidence level, cited in a meta-analysis of randomized controlled trial (RCT) clinical studies

Why Did I Write this Book?

Like most women who turn 50, I was advised by my doctor to get a baseline BMD (bone mineral density) test. She actually had a separate bone density clinic next door to her OB/GYN practice, run by a partner physician. How convenient, I thought.

I scheduled my appointment. When I went in to have the BMD test, the DXA (Dual-Energy X-ray Absorptiometry, formerly called DEXA) scan was easy and painless. After I left, I realized that I didn't know as much as I needed to know about the whole subject of bone health. As a health researcher, I knew that I would be unwilling to just accept whatever the doctor might tell me about it when I went back for my results.

It isn't that I distrust doctors – it's that I know that they are very busy. To start with, they have problems that we can only thank our lucky stars that we will never face. They leave medical school with astronomical student loan debt to repay.

To protect themselves from lawsuits devastating them financially, they are forced to carry malpractice insurance with huge premiums that take another chunk of their profits. So practicing medicine isn't nearly as lucrative as the general public seems to think it is.

Not only are physicians loaded with all of these enormous upfront costs of doing business, but they also have to contend with real barriers to giving people the best medical care – care that they can feel good about having provided. Health insurance companies, particularly those designated HMO (Health Management Organization), are calling the shots when it comes to what your doctor can and cannot do for you.

By setting up limits on which tests or surgical procedures will (or will not) be paid for or at what rate, or how much the prescription cost for each medication will be according to their formulary, they significantly influence how medicine is practiced by physicians today. In fact, in almost every meaningful way, insurance companies are the ones that are effectively practicing medicine now, instead of the doctors.

Truly, you could not pay me enough to be a doctor, given the current conditions under which they operate. I am very glad that people do want to become doctors, especially surgeons. If I had an accident that required surgery to save my life, I would be ever grateful that there are surgeons that could do so.

Add to all of this enormous stress that doctors are dealing with every day, the need to herd as many patients as possible through their offices as quickly as possible every day, just to meet the financial burdens placed upon them by the student loans and malpractice insurance. Doctors probably have less free time at their disposal than almost any other profession. I doubt that many doctors find enough time to spend with their families, much less find the time to do any research. No wonder they are being educated by pharmaceutical reps.

And if the drug company reps are providing the information, it's no wonder that doctors rely more on a pill or other drug than on any other type of treatment for any condition. It's what they know about. Of course, what they know is what the drug companies want them to know—and usually nothing else.

The net result of all of this is that doctors end up telling us lies – not lies that they know that they are telling, but lies of which they are entirely unaware. For this reason, I always do my own health research – and my research into osteoporosis was particularly enlightening.

When I got the call from the nurse telling me that the test showed that I had osteopenia (normal thinning of the bones caused by aging), and that I needed to come back for a consult with the doctor, I asked her what the doctor would want me to do. She told me that he would likely want me to take Actonel to protect my bones from further thinning.

I was able to tell her confidently that there was no need for me to come in for that consult, then, because the very last thing that I would ever do to improve my bone health would be to take a bisphosphonate like Actonel, because I knew it would only make things worse over time.

She gasped.

16

Get the Facts

Part 1

Psychoanalyst **Walter Langer** wrote:

"People will believe a big lie sooner than a little one. And if you repeat it frequently enough, people will sooner than later believe it."

Most physicians will tell you to do four things to reduce your risk of breaking bones as you age:

1. Take bisphosphonate drugs.

2. Take calcium supplements.

3. Do weight-bearing exercises.

4. And if your doctor has heard about the newer tests to determine Vitamin D deficiency, that awareness might mean that you get tested and possibly prescribed supplemental Vitamin D.

This just might be some of the worst advice that you have ever been given.

Here's why:

1. Bisphosphonate drugs can actually increase your risk of fractures over time, as well as subject you to dangerous, potentially disfiguring side effects, such as the death of your jawbone. No one is telling you this.

2. Calcium supplements taken alone can increase your risk of calcification of the arteries.

3. Weight-bearing exercises, done in the wrong way, will not strengthen bones as much as a new type of workout that also optimizes your hormonal responses. Other newer technologies also exist that allow those unable to do much movement to benefit.

4. Vitamin D supplements, even prescriptions, if they are not the correct type, will not help your bone health. And too much can be toxic without Vitamin A.

What do I suggest instead?

17

1. Take Vitamin K2 (<u>always with Vitamin D3 [or 15-20 minutes of sunshine] and Vitamin A</u>), especially if taking calcium supplements.

2. Reduce or eliminate the drugs you are taking that can endanger your bone health, such as SSRIs, certain popular blood thinners such as warfarin (Coumadin), and even GERD (acid reflux) medications.

3. Get adequate sleep, at least 6 hours, preferably 8 hours, which is a real problem for many today.

4. Get adequate sun (15-20 minutes a day) **without sunscreen** or if that is impossible, take Vitamin D in the optimal form, D3, but only with Vitamin A also.

Fact: Taking calcium without Vitamin K2 leads to calcification of arteries. Vitamin K2 affects calcium regulation through carboxylation of a protein called osteocalcin. Carboxylated osteocalcin helps to direct calcium in the body into the bones and teeth, rather than into the blood vessels as atherosclerosis or in other inappropriate locations such as bone spurs causing arthritis.

By carboxylating and therefore activating the Matrix GLA Proteins (MGPs) in the body (responsible for cleaning the arteries of calcium deposits in plaques), K2 can actually reverse the calcification that is already present in soft tissues.

In one study, a 37-50% decrease in calcification took place. http://www.ncbi.nlm.nih.gov/pubmed/17138823 Abstract http://bloodjournal.hematologylibrary.org/content/109/7/2 823.full.pdf Full Article —Note that this amazing 50% clearing of calcium from the arteries took place in only six weeks. http://www.ncbi.nlm.nih.gov/pubmed/14654717 http://www.ncbi.nlm.nih.gov/pubmed/19179058 http://www.ncbi.nlm.nih.gov/pubmed/11374034 http://www.ncbi.nlm.nih.gov/pubmed/22692665 http://www.ncbi.nlm.nih.gov/pubmed/21088475 http://www.ncbi.nlm.nih.gov/pubmed/9743228 http://www.ncbi.nlm.nih.gov/pubmed/21775389 http://www.ncbi.nlm.nih.gov/pubmed/20354170 http://www.ncbi.nlm.nih.gov/pubmed/24285428 http://www.ncbi.nlm.nih.gov/pubmed/18234293 http://www.ncbi.nlm.nih.gov/pubmed/18196985

http://www.ncbi.nlm.nih.gov/pubmed/16030366
http://www.ncbi.nlm.nih.gov/pubmed/15775408
http://www.ncbi.nlm.nih.gov/pubmed/14961167
http://www.ncbi.nlm.nih.gov/pubmed/10806559

Fact: Warfarin (Coumadin) depletes Vitamin K2 and causes arterial calcification. Many physicians are unaware of how extremely detrimental that long-term (more than 6 months) Coumadin use can be for both bones and heart because:

- It prevents proper bone formation due to its effects on Vitamin K2 levels (owing to its blocking Vitamin K epoxide reductase to reduce the clotting factors normally made in the liver, thereby also blocking the ability to recycle Vitamin K).
- It simultaneously worsens arterial wall rupture risks (since calcification of the arteries can result from K2 deficiency, especially when taking calcium supplements).

They only prescribe warfarin because it is old and familiar to them, with no alternatives being available until recently. Adequate levels of Vitamin K2 are vital to both proper bone-building and cardiovascular health.
http://www.ncbi.nlm.nih.gov/pubmed/22952653
http://www.ncbi.nlm.nih.gov/pubmed/22520397
http://www.ncbi.nlm.nih.gov/pubmed/17598002
http://www.ncbi.nlm.nih.gov/pubmed/17138823
http://www.ncbi.nlm.nih.gov/pubmed/17598002
http://www.ncbi.nlm.nih.gov/pubmed/22169620
http://www.ncbi.nlm.nih.gov/pubmed/18722618
http://www.ncbi.nlm.nih.gov/pubmed/15514282
http://www.ncbi.nlm.nih.gov/pubmed/24072176
http://www.ncbi.nlm.nih.gov/pubmed/19793187

In 2004 and 2005, studies of over 100 subjects showed that those taking vitamin K-blocking anticoagulants have twice the calcification of those not on these drugs.
http://www.ncbi.nlm.nih.gov/pubmed/15265793
http://www.ncbi.nlm.nih.gov/pubmed/16169351

Many patients with a history of atrial fibrillation, transient ischemic attack (TIA or mini-stroke) or cerebrovascular accident (CVA or stroke) are treated with blood thinners in an effort to prevent further cardiovascular events. Most are given Vitamin K depleting drugs such as warfarin (Coumadin) because it is well-known and has been used for a long time. However, it is not necessary to use that type of blood thinner (anticoagulant), since there are different types available now.

Many anticoagulants inhibit FactorXa (activated coagulant Factor X) activity. Some of them do it indirectly through binding to circulating antithrombin, which is abbreviated AT III. These are the injected anticoagulants, such as unfractionated heparin (UFH), low molecular weight heparin (LMWH), and fondaparinux. These cannot be taken orally, as they are inactive in an oral form.

Other anticoagulants, the so-called VKAs (Vitamin K antagonists), reduce the synthesis in the liver of many coagulation factors, including Factor Xa. Included in this class of anticoagulants are the popular drugs warfarin (Coumadin), phenprocoumon, and acenocoumarol, which are still effective when taken orally. Be aware that warfarin (Coumadin) is also commonly used as rat poison.

Fact: Warfarin (Coumadin) depletes Vitamin K2 and causes increased thinning of bones.
http://www.ncbi.nlm.nih.gov/pubmed/9412619

Fact: Alternatives to Coumadin exist now. Newer oral, direct acting inhibitors of Factor Xa have entered clinical development and some are already available. These include rivaroxaban (Xarelto), apixaban, betrixaban, LY517717, darexaban (YM150), and DU-176b edoxaban. Dabigatran is a direct thrombin inhibitor. Replacing Coumadin with either Pradaxa, Xarelto (rivaroxaban), or a combination of Lovenox and aspirin is the best option.

After this has been done, patients can replenish their K2 levels to potentially completely reverse the damage by beginning to take Vitamin K2, preferably menaquinone-4, known as MK-4. That side of the chain has better bone effects and the additional advantage that it can augment the beta cells in the pancreas, so it's particularly preferred for Type 2 diabetics over the other forms, including MK-7.

http://www.ncbi.nlm.nih.gov/pubmed/14654717

However, MK-7 is easier to dose because its half-life is longer than MK-4's, meaning that it can be taken less often because it remains in the body longer. Half-life is the amount of time it takes the body to excrete half of the substance.

Toxicity studies show that up to 10mg per kg of body weight was considered safe, and the NOAEL (No Observed Adverse Effect Level) of MK-7 over a 90-day period of oral administration to rats was 10mg per kg of body weight per day, which was the highest dose tested, so no toxicity level has been found yet.
http://www.ncbi.nlm.nih.gov/pubmed/21781006
http://toxnet.nlm.nih.gov/cgi-bin/sis/search/a?dbs+hsdb:@term+@DOCNO+1040

However, about 30% of the population with certain genotypes (APOE polymorphisms) might not excrete MK-7 or even MK-4 as fast as the rest of us, although the study results have lacked consensus. Anecdotal reports (not clinical studies, just someone's story) of arrhythmias with taking too much MK-7 can be found on the internet. The MK-7 form of K2 can cause insomnia and/or rapid heartbeat in doses over 100 mcg.
http://advances.nutrition.org/content/3/2/182.full

As for safety regarding risk for blood clots, the risk does not increase even with extremely high doses, at least for MK-4, which was the form used in the studies with humans. Up to 45 mg per day were tested.
http://www.ncbi.nlm.nih.gov/pubmed/11846334
http://dx.doi.org/10.1016/S0378-5122(01)00275-4

In rat studies, doses as high as 250 mg/kg of body weight did not increase blood-clotting, nor the blood platelet aggregation rate. http://dx.doi.org/10.1016/S0021-9150(97)00087-7

TAT and F1+2 are sensitive molecular markers that reflect thrombin amounts in the blood. In 2001, a study of 29 elderly patients showed no changes in these markers while on MK-4 K2 treatment.
http://www.ncbi.nlm.nih.gov/pubmed/11846334

But what about those taking warfarin (Coumadin) for a condition requiring anti-coagulation drugs? Can they take K2 without risk of increasing coagulation?

An interesting question indeed, one that is being explored by researchers who reported in 2005 that the common practice of restricting Vitamin K dietary intake while taking warfarin could be the worst thing to do in order to stabilize INR (International Normalized Ratio), which is a measure of normalized coagulation time. Patients on anticoagulation therapy are monitored to be sure that their INR remains stable within a therapeutic range that does not put them at high risk for either blood clots (lower INR) or bleeding (higher INR). Dosage is adjusted to attempt to keep the patient within the safest range possible.

Patients were divided into two groups, 26 whose INR had been stable for 6 months, and 26 whose INR had been unstable during that period. The stable patients averaged 76 mcg per day of Vitamin K dietary intake while the unstable ones averaged only 29 mcg per day.

After considering the fact that increasing daily intake of Vitamin K by 100 mcg per day only reduces INR by .2, a very small effect, the researchers' conclusion was that daily Vitamin K supplementation might be a better approach to achieving stable anticoagulation control, by decreasing the impact of dietary intake (which can and does vary considerably on a daily basis) on INR stability. However, the Vitamin K used in that study was K1, whereas K2 would be the preferred form, according to Cees Vermeer, leading Vitamin K expert, in his response to this study, which also points out that K1 would not protect against calcification. If that K2 is MK-7, it has 3 to 4 times the effect on INR, however.
http://www.bloodjournal.org/content/109/8/3279
http://www.ncbi.nlm.nih.gov/pubmed/14717783
http://www.ncbi.nlm.nih.gov/pubmed/17110451
http://www.ncbi.nlm.nih.gov/pubmed/15886802
http://www.bloodjournal.org/content/109/8/3607.1

Other proponents of a low-dose daily intake of Vitamin K2 to stabilize INR in those being treating with anticoagulants

include Johannes Oldenburg, a medical research scientist who believes it could reduce risk of bleeding issues.
http://www.ncbi.nlm.nih.gov/pubmed/15886790

If someone did want to take K2 while taking a Vitamin K antagonist like warfarin, their INR would need to be monitored closely by their health provider until it was at a desired stable level.

Another concern with K2 supplements is the fact that natural K2 MK-4 is the "trans" form, while synthetic K2 MK-4 might contain some of the unnatural "cis" form, which could theoretically have a different effect on the body.

The MK-7 form builds up in the body, whereas MK-4 cannot, due to the fact that MK-4 only has a half-life of 3-4 hours, but MK-7 has a 3.5 day half-life.

All of the studies to date showing prevention of fractures have been done with MK-4, not MK-7, so we do not know if MK-7 would be an acceptable substitute for MK-4 in terms of strengthening bones. Studies show that MK-7 can carboxylate osteocalcin (OC), but does it do the same for Matrix GLA Protein (MGP)? Two of the newer studies indicate that it does, since administration of MK-7 caused uncarboxylated MGP levels to decrease just as uncarboxylated OC levels did.
http://www.ncbi.nlm.nih.gov/pubmed/22169620
http://www.ncbi.nlm.nih.gov/pubmed/23062766

A 2013 study showed that MK-7 increased bone mineral density and strengthened bones:
http://www.ncbi.nlm.nih.gov/pubmed/23525894

Taking both MK-7 and MK-4 might be ideal if a Vitamin K2 deficiency exists, since they do have some different effects from each other, with MK-4 having better bone effects and can enhance the beta cells in the pancreas for diabetics, while MK-7 has a more potent effect on cardiovascular health by better inhibiting calcification, although taking either one is better than taking none. This is the only product with both together:
http://www.amazon.com/dp/B004GW4S0G

Fact: A patent application was filed in 2011 by a large drug company for a timed-release type of Vitamin K2 to treat osteoporosis.
http://tinyurl.com/K2Patent

Fact: In 1995, the Ministry of Health in Japan approved this treatment for osteoporosis. According to the Archives of Internal Medicine, taking a daily dose of 45 mg of K2 in the form of MK-4:
- decreased all non-spinal fractures by 81%
- decreased broken hips by 77%
- decreased spinal fracture risk by 60%

Health claims are allowed for one K2 supplement already on the market in Japan, based on positive studies.
http://www.ncbi.nlm.nih.gov/pubmed/16801507
http://www.ncbi.nlm.nih.gov/pubmed/10874601
http://www.ncbi.nlm.nih.gov/pubmed/17012826
http://www.ncbi.nlm.nih.gov/pubmed/22392526
http://www.ncbi.nlm.nih.gov/pubmed/22301331
http://www.ncbi.nlm.nih.gov/pubmed/21295170
http://www.ncbi.nlm.nih.gov/pubmed/15664003

Fact: The preferred treatment for osteoporosis in Japan is Vitamin K2. Vitamin K2 aids normal coagulation of blood, while avoiding the potential excessive clotting when used in high doses that could be seen with Vitamin K1. Menatetrenone, also known as MK-4, is a Vitamin K2 menaquinone compound marketed for osteoporosis in Japan by Eisai Co., under the trade name Glakay.
http://www.ncbi.nlm.nih.gov/pubmed/17287908
http://www.ncbi.nlm.nih.gov/pubmed/9737352
http://www.ncbi.nlm.nih.gov/pubmed/10457281
http://www.drugweb.net/Eisai/drug/menatetrenone/Glakay/Osteoporosis/Japan/

Fact: NASA uses K2 to protect astronauts from bone loss while in microgravity in space.
http://www.ncbi.nlm.nih.gov/pubmed/12361778
http://www.ncbi.nlm.nih.gov/pubmed/11316009
http://www.ncbi.nlm.nih.gov/pubmed/16077253

Chickens are Being Protected from Fractures Better than You Are

Fact: The feed of chickens and other poultry, as well as pigs, contains Vitamin K, the purpose of which is to strengthen their bones. Even though it is a rather toxic synthetic form called menadione, because the animals can synthesize menaquinone-4 (MK-4) from it, they are protected from fractures during transport because of this feed additive.

Although I am fully aware that mere "association" or "correlation" does not necessarily equate to "causation," it is worth mentioning that both longevity and fewer cardiovascular events, as well as less cancer incidence, have been shown to be correlated or associated with taking K2.

Fact: Taking K2 is associated with living longer.
The first study demonstrating the beneficial effect of Vitamin K2, the Rotterdam Study, showed that the life expectancy of those who had 45 mcg of K2 intake was seven years longer than those in the lowest quartile, and that was 12 mcg per day.
http://www.ncbi.nlm.nih.gov/pubmed/15514282

Fact: Taking K2 is associated with less cancer.
http://www.ncbi.nlm.nih.gov/pubmed/20335553
http://www.ncbi.nlm.nih.gov/pubmed/12946240
http://www.ncbi.nlm.nih.gov/pubmed/15703828

Fact: Taking more K2 is correlated with fewer cardiovascular events. Subsequently, the Prospect study was an independent 10-year-long study of 16,000 subjects that calculated that for each 10 mcg K2 in the diet, these people had 9% fewer cardiovascular events, which would come out to 40% less risk for 45 mcg.
http://www.ncbi.nlm.nih.gov/pubmed/19179058

Fact: If you are taking an SSRI (selective serotonin reuptake inhibitor) type of antidepressant, such as Cymbalta, Paxil, Prozac, and many others, which affects circulating serotonin levels in the gut, your body's bone building regulation is disrupted as well. The gut hormonally controls bone formation using signaling from the serotonin stored in the enterochromaffin (EC) cells of the gut lining, which is the majority of all serotonin in the body, meaning that serotonin is really a gut hormone related to bone building, as well as a neurotransmitter in the brain.

Fact: DXA scans can only give BMD results. BMD does not measure bone quality, only density. Low BMD alone as an effective predictor of elevated fracture risk, although commonly used in clinical practice as the gold standard, is not considered proven, only "associated" with fracture risk, and is in fact debated as an effective predictor of fracture among medical community members, as this link to an article in the peer-reviewed medical journal *Bone* shows.
DXA in vivo BMD methodology: an erroneous and misleading research and clinical gauge of bone mineral status, bone fragility, and bone remodelling.
http://www.ncbi.nlm.nih.gov/pubmed/17481978
http://www.ncbi.nlm.nih.gov/pubmed/12817754

Fact: DXA scans and BMD are used mainly because no other alternatives exist to induce compliance with osteoporosis treatment. To get you to take the drugs, these tests must be used as justification. In fact, one section states that two randomized controlled trials (RCTs) and seven published meta-analyses of RCTs concerning BMD monitoring during osteoporosis therapy proved that although higher increases in BMD were generally associated with reduced risk of fracture, only a small percentage of the fracture risk reduction could be explained by BMD and some experienced significant fracture risk reduction with little or no increase in BMD.

Despite this non-correlation between BMD and fracture reduction, the study stated that BMD is still the only test available for monitoring responses to osteoporosis therapy. In the Conclusion, it adds that BMD is the only tool available to help motivate patients to continue treatment, and to advise the patient that it could take longer than a year to get results and to continue treatment even in absence of response or even when bone loss is seen; but in this case, question whether the patient is taking the medication properly or not.
http://www.ncbi.nlm.nih.gov/pmc/articles/PMC3379167/
http://www.ncbi.nlm.nih.gov/pubmed/23074491

http://www.medscape.com/viewarticle/782730

Fact: The pooled clinical fracture reduction for bisphosphonates was only 22% in a 2010 cross-design synthesis review. Better (and safer) results can be obtained with alternatives in the form of Vitamin K2, Vitamin D3, Vitamin A, and other natural supplements that I will share with you. Taking serious side-effect risks simply isn't necessary to protect your bones.
http://www.ncbi.nlm.nih.gov/pubmed/19572092

Fact: Taking bisphosphonates does not make bones stronger, only thicker, and the actual bone quality diminishes over time, the longer the drugs are taken. Since 1995, when the FDA approved the first bisphosphonate as an osteoporosis drug, women who have been advised to take such a drug have been sold a bill of goods for which the piper now wants to be paid. And the price is high.

Fact: Bisphosphonates carry the risk of serious side effects. Many clinical studies exist to show these:
http://www.ncbi.nlm.nih.gov/pubmed/23838024
http://www.ncbi.nlm.nih.gov/pubmed/24177063
http://www.ncbi.nlm.nih.gov/pubmed/19570737
http://www.ncbi.nlm.nih.gov/pubmed/21504254
http://www.ncbi.nlm.nih.gov/pubmed/20173017
http://www.ncbi.nlm.nih.gov/pubmed/23858334
http://www.ncbi.nlm.nih.gov/pubmed/23921518
http://www.ncbi.nlm.nih.gov/pubmed/24150190
http://www.ncbi.nlm.nih.gov/pubmed/23184667
http://www.ncbi.nlm.nih.gov/pubmed/23332469
http://www.ncbi.nlm.nih.gov/pubmed/23296595
http://www.ncbi.nlm.nih.gov/pubmed/23315281
http://www.ncbi.nlm.nih.gov/pubmed/22732749
http://www.ncbi.nlm.nih.gov/pubmed/22691683
http://www.ncbi.nlm.nih.gov/pubmed/22753670
http://www.ncbi.nlm.nih.gov/pubmed/19066707
http://www.ncbi.nlm.nih.gov/pubmed/17663640

Serious Side Effects of Bisphosphonates

Let's discuss some of the more serious side effects in more detail, the first of them being the most ironic imaginable.

Atypical Femoral Fractures

A new acronym is appearing in the medical journals more and more frequently: AFF (Atypical Femoral Fractures).

Following is an X-ray image showing an AFF that occurred after 63 months of alendronate (generic of Fosamax) therapy.

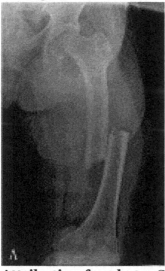

Out of 310 cases of atypical femoral fractures, task force researchers found a shocking 94% of them had been using bisphosphonates for at least five years, reported a study published by the *Journal of Bone and Mineral Research*.

http://www.ncbi.nlm.nih.gov/pubmed/25538222
http://www.ncbi.nlm.nih.gov/pubmed/25495429
http://www.ncbi.nlm.nih.gov/pubmed/20842676
http://www.ncbi.nlm.nih.gov/pubmed/23216704
http://www.ncbi.nlm.nih.gov/pubmed/22730621
http://www.ncbi.nlm.nih.gov/pubmed/20809164
http://www.ncbi.nlm.nih.gov/pubmed/23748615
http://www.ncbi.nlm.nih.gov/pubmed/23426763

One 59-year-old, who had been taking Fosamax for 8 years, was jumping rope with children in her neighborhood, when suddenly, her thighbone snapped in two at the bottom of one hop. What a traumatic experience — not only for her, but for the unfortunate children who witnessed their neighbor's agony and bewilderment — no doubt feeling completely helpless to stop what was probably the worst pain they'd ever seen anyone suffer. Maybe I'm all wrong here, but wouldn't breaking the largest bone in your body — not just a crack, but broken completely in two — be the very last thing that you would expect to happen to you after years of taking medication that your doctor assured you would lessen your chances of breaking bones?
http://abcnews.go.com/GMA/OnCall/fosamax-long-term-bone-strengthening-drug-linked-fractures/story?id=10045179

Finally, the FDA released a statement about increased fracture risk when using bisphosphonates for longer than five years, although studies were already validating the experiences of patients reported in the news much earlier.

It took from March 2010 to September 2011 for the FDA to take action to inform the public. And the statement only said that it would be safe to discontinue after 3 to 4 years, but did not explain the increased fracture risks if it was continued.
http://www.fda.gov/downloads/AdvisoryCommittees/CommitteesMeetingMaterials/Drugs/DrugSafetyandRiskManagementAdvisoryCommittee/UCM270958.pdf

Your risk of fractures actually increases the longer that you take it, because almost every osteoporosis drug on the market works by increasing bone density without enhancing bone quality. Good bone quality means that you won't break a bone if you fall, because your bone has the right connective tissue and minerals complex necessary to allow you to absorb the impact instead of fracturing, if the bone is strong and flexible. This is the way that Vitamin K2 works, by stimulating formation of connective tissue in bone, which strengthens bone quality, the true desired outcome to save yourself from a fracture.

After two years of bisphosphonate treatment, almost no new remineralized surfaces exist in the bones for all dosages, less than 1%, versus 7.57% new mineralization for those not on the treatment. http://www.ncbi.nlm.nih.gov/pubmed/9294113

Keep that fact in mind while you read this sad story from a medical journal case report from Singapore in which a woman took alendronate for osteopenia. She didn't even have osteoporosis. One year later, she developed a stress fracture and discontinued the drug. After it healed, 3 years later, she had a normal BMD.

Five years later, for some reason that was not explained, her oncologist gave her ibandronate, another bisphosphonate. After 7 months, she fell and broke both femurs completely in two – bilateral simultaneous displaced fractures. Follow the link to see the horrifying X-ray in Figure 3, which really tells this story best.
http://www.ncbi.nlm.nih.gov/pmc/articles/PMC3235321/

A picture really is worth a thousand words, isn't it?

Osteonecrosis of the Jaw

In fact, there is now an acronym created for this side effect: BRONJ (Bisphosphonate-Related Osteonecrosis of the Jaw) http://www.ncbi.nlm.nih.gov/pubmed/25549869

According to a June 2012 article in the *Journal of Evidence-Based Dental Practice,* your risk of other irreversible serious side effects such as jaw bone death also increases severely after two years.
http://www.ncbi.nlm.nih.gov/pubmed/22726797

In fact, according to a 2007 University of British Columbia study, the risk is almost tripled. "Popular Osteoporosis Drugs Triple Risk of Painful Bone Necrosis, Study Finds."
http://www.sciencedaily.com/releases/2008/01/080115092048.htm
The underlying clinical study is available here:
http://jrheum.org/content/35/4/691.abstract

BRONJ occurrences increased from 1.5% in those on bisphosphonates for a year or less, to 7.7% in those exposed to them for more than three years. Higher risk factors included dental procedures and a specific bisphosphonate, zoledronic acid.
http://www.ncbi.nlm.nih.gov/pubmed/16314620

The American Society for Bone and Mineral Research formed a task force to research and report on the association of ONJ with bisphosphonate therapy.
http://www.ncbi.nlm.nih.gov/pubmed/17663640

How would you feel if you could no longer eat solid food or speak clearly, all because you wanted to have strong bones? The Prolia TV commercial mentions severe jawbone problems. What they don't mention is that it involves the necrosis or DEATH of the jawbone, which can have permanently disfiguring consequences and is NOT a temporary minor inconvenience.

This disease of the jaw first surfaced in match factories, where workers contracted what was called at the time "phossy jaw" because they were handling phosphorus during the manufacture of the head of the matches, which were made of white phosphorus at the time. Matches are now made with red phosphorous to prevent this condition in factories.
http://www.ncbi.nlm.nih.gov/pubmed/18940506

Thanks to the FDA and drug manufacturers, we are seeing a resurgence of this disease since osteoporosis treatment began using bisphosphonates, which are alarmingly similar to the chemical that white phosphorous became after absorption into the body.

And what if you get an infected tooth that needs to be pulled? If you need dental work and have been on these drugs for any amount of time at all, dentists will not do the work if it involves pulling teeth or dental surgery of any kind, because of the threat of jaw necrosis.

Unfortunately, you only find this out after the fact, when you discover that you can't get the dental care that you need because of having taken these osteoporosis drugs. Dentists know well the risks of bisphosphonates, even if your prescribing doctor does not, and most will not take the risk to treat you, due to the liability that they would be taking on.

The American Dental Association states that their study shows 4% of people on bisphosphonates developed BRONJ. http://www.ada.org/3130.aspx

Atrial Fibrillation

In 2013, a fast, irregular heartbeat was being associated with bisphosphonate use. A meta-analysis by Maimonides Medical Center in New York of randomized controlled studies showed that the risk of serious atrial fibrillation (A-Fib) requiring hospitalization was increased by 40% in bisphosphonate users. http://www.ncbi.nlm.nih.gov/pubmed/23722644

Note that this is in obvious disagreement with the FDA announcement on November, 12, 2008, that they saw no clear relationship between bisphosphonate use and A-Fib when they reviewed the clinical trials. Their recommendation? No alterations in prescribing for health care professionals, nor cessation of treatment for patients. http://www.fda.gov./cder/drug/early_comm/bisphosphona tes_update_200811.htm

Esophageal Cancer

The results are not so clear-cut when it comes to the possibility of increased esophageal cancer risk, though. The studies are so conflicting that a definitive link cannot be assumed. http://www.ncbi.nlm.nih.gov/pubmed/22333262

Risk found:
http://www.ncbi.nlm.nih.gov/pubmed/20813820

http://www.ncbi.nlm.nih.gov/pubmed/22966908
http://www.ncbi.nlm.nih.gov/pubmed/12184516
http://meetinglibrary.asco.org/content/92963-114

No Risk found:
http://www.ncbi.nlm.nih.gov/pubmed/23052941
http://www.ncbi.nlm.nih.gov/pubmed/23155320
http://www.ncbi.nlm.nih.gov/pubmed/23325866
http://www.ncbi.nlm.nih.gov/pubmed/20699457

Perhaps the answer is that prolonged bisphosphonate use is needed to see a significant link.
http://www.ncbi.nlm.nih.gov/pubmed/21537362

There is an increased, though not actually statistically significant, risk of esophageal cancer in long-term users of oral bisphosphonates.
http://www.ncbi.nlm.nih.gov/pmc/articles/PMC3484348/

In a letter to the New England Journal of Medicine in 2009, a doctor outlined 23 instances of esophageal cancer reported to the FDA during 1995-2008, for which oral bisphosphonates were suspected as being possible tumor promoters. The median time from drug use to diagnosis was 2.1 years in the United States and 1.3 years in Europe and Japan. The physician that wrote this letter also recommended that patients with Barrett's esophagus should not be prescribed bisphosphonates.
http://www.ncbi.nlm.nih.gov/pubmed/19118315

Renal Toxicity

Another serious potential risk for bisphosphonate use is that of renal toxicity, which means a risk for kidney failure. Studies that show this link are numerous.
http://www.ncbi.nlm.nih.gov/pubmed/16313549
http://www.ncbi.nlm.nih.gov/pubmed/17491196
http://www.ncbi.nlm.nih.gov/pubmed/12787420
http://www.ncbi.nlm.nih.gov/pubmed/19013118
http://www.ncbi.nlm.nih.gov/pubmed/19581797
http://www.ncbi.nlm.nih.gov/pubmed/16364053

Musculoskeletal Pain

The FDA issued an alert on January 7, 2008, about the "possibility of severe and sometimes incapacitating bone, joint, and/or muscle (musculoskeletal) pain in patients taking bisphosphonates. The severe musculoskeletal pain may occur within days, months or years after starting a bisphosphonate. Some patients have reported complete relief of symptoms after discontinuing the bisphosphonate, whereas others have reported slow or incomplete resolution. This severe musculoskeletal pain is in contrast to the acute phase response characterized by fever, chills, bone pain, myalgias, and arthralgias that sometimes accompany initial administration of intravenous bisphosphonates and may occur with initial exposure to once-weekly or once-monthly doses of oral bisphosphonates. The symptoms related to the acute phase response tend to resolve within several days with continuing drug use."

http://www.fda.gov/cder/drug/infopage/bisphosphonates/default.htm

This alert was in response to 116 adverse event reports received for alendronate and 6 for risedronate between 1995 and 2002.

Calcitonin: Fish-Based, and Fishy, But Not Banned in the US Yet

Natural-sounding alternatives to bisphosphonates might not be safe to use, either. Calcitonin (synthetic recombinant DNA nasal spray forms are named Miacalcin and Fortical), sometimes referred to as calcitonin salmon because the nasal mist, injection, or pill is fish-based, was approved by the FDA in 1988.

Almost 25 years later, an internal FDA memo released ahead of an FDA panel meeting stated that "the potential for a cancer risk with calcitonin salmon therapy cannot be ignored. The majority of all calcitonin salmon trials showed an increased risk estimate." And even the makers admit that they have never known the means by which it might work.

Initially, the FDA had approved the drugs based on studies that showed increased bone mineral density in users. The most notable fact about this FDA panel's recommendation is that they stated that no studies have definitively shown that higher bone density really reduces risk of bone fractures, and therefore, the drug cannot be said to be effective to prevent fractures. And by far the most interesting fact about that is that the very same thing can be said about the most often prescribed drugs for osteoporosis today, bisphosphonates.

Although the vote to no longer recommend calcitonin as an osteoporosis drug was 12 to 9, the same FDA panel voted 20 to 1 that any future calcitonin drugs should be required to show real effectiveness in preventing bone fractures.

However, the FDA is not required in any way to follow the recommendations of its own panels, and this one was no exception. The October 2013 publication of the conclusion of a review of all the studies regarding calcitonin might have been expected to finally spur the FDA to take action, but it did not: http://aop.sagepub.com/content/47/12/1675

Canada Health banned calcitonin October 1, 2013.
http://globalnews.ca/news/753964/calcitonin-nasal-sprays-to-be-pulled-from-market-due-to-cancer-risk/

Unsurprisingly, over one year earlier, in July 2012, the European Medicines Agency had ruled that calcitonin should no longer be used to treat osteoporosis because of the drug's cancer risk, which they stated varied between 0.7% in studies with the oral calcitonin-containing formulation to 2.4% in the studies with the nasal calcitonin-containing formulation. http://www.ema.europa.eu/ema/index.jsp?curl=pages/medicines/human/referrals/Calcitonin/human_referral_000319.jsp&mid=WC0b01ac0580024e99

A review of randomized controlled trials for salmon calcitonin use and associated cancer risk was published December 2013. http://www.ncbi.nlm.nih.gov/pubmed/24259626

The Taiwanese FDA banned calcitonin on December 1, 2013. http://www.chinapost.com.tw/taiwan/national/national-news/2013/11/30/394862/FDA-orders.htm

What did the US FDA finally do? Not much. In March, 2014, it changed the nasal mist label and injection prescribing insert to include a warning about the increased cancer risk: http://www.fda.gov/Safety/MedWatch/SafetyInformation/ucm190771.htm http://www.accessdata.fda.gov/drugsatfda_docs/label/2014/017808s035lbl.pdf

Calcitonin is still approved for use in the US.

Why Isn't The FDA Protecting Me From These Drugs?

Well, a change was made in how the FDA is funded, in 1992. After 86 years during which the FDA funding came from the US Treasury, like other government agencies, the fox is truly watching the henhouse now. The large pharmaceutical companies are paying fees to the FDA, supposedly to allow America to get drugs approved faster than before, but the intention of the fees is not how it is in practice.

As you might expect, this relationship has become incestuous, with executives moving freely back and forth between the FDA and pharmaceutical or medication companies (or their law firms) for employment. Just do an internet search for Keith Webber, Dr. Lawrence Yu, Chang H. Ahn, Dr. Mark McClellan, Daniel E. Troy, and Ralph Tyler. Or check out: http://www.cptech.org/ip/health/politics/revolvingdoor.html

Medications that are Harmful to Your Bones

Part 2

"First, do no harm."

Nearly every drug that you see advertised on television is damaging to your skeletal health, not to mention your overall health in general. That's right, if Big Pharma is spending big bucks to tell you to ask your doctor if "x" drug is "right for you," it probably isn't.

Big Pharma won't rest until every person on the earth is taking the following recipe for disaster:
- Cholesterol Lowering Statins: Lipitor, Plavix
- Antidepressants: Cymbalta, Abilify
- Acid Reflux and GERD: Nexium, Prilosec, Zantac
- High Blood Pressure medications: Lisinopril
- Bisphosphonates and other drugs for Osteoporosis: Boniva, Actonel, Atelvia, Fosamax, Binosto, Reclast, Aclasta, Forteo, Evista, Protelos, Miacalcin, Fortical
- Erectile dysfunction medications (men only): Cialis, Viagra

And they will tell you that you won't be healthy unless you take them all, for the rest of your life.

And they will continue to lobby the medical establishment to lower the numbers required to be considered in healthy ranges, in order to force more and more people into the range that requires medication.

Remember when perfect blood pressure was 120 over 80? Well, it isn't anymore. Beginning in 2003 with The Seventh Report of the Joint National Committee on Prevention, Detection, Evaluation, and Treatment of High Blood Pressure, if your BP was 120/80, you are now told that it is "pre-hypertensive" or a level that might require meds to lower. And for every 10 points that these levels can be lowered, the drug companies make millions more as thousands more are added to the list of their customers.

Osteoporosis Drugs

Surprise! Perhaps the most potentially harmful drug for bone health is in the very class of drugs that your doctor will want you to take to increase your BMD (bone mineral density). These drugs include:

- Bisphosphonates:
  - o Actonel (Risedronic acid or risedronate) and Atelvia (risedronate combined with a delayed-release coating to eliminate fasting required by other bisphosphonates)
  - o Fosamax (Alendronic acid / alendronate sodium) or Binosto (an effervescent version of Fosamax)
  - o Boniva (Ibandronic acid or ibandronate)
  - o Reclast or Zometa (zoledronic acid, marketed as Aclasta outside the US) is the once-yearly injectable bisphosphonate. It is also used as chemotherapy for cancer treatment.
- Evista (Raloxifene, a SERM [selective estrogen receptor modulator], which acts on estrogen receptors in selected tissues through simulating the hormone) and recently approved Duavee (Conjugated estrogens [similar to Premarin] combined with a SERM, bazedoxifene.) The mechanism of action is similar to that of HRT for mimicking estrogen to inhibit osteoclast activity in order to decrease bone resorption.
- Prolia (Denosumab) is an injected laboratory-made antibody that binds to RANK Ligand to reduce osteoclast differentiation, activity and survival, which leads to a decrease in bone resorption.
- Forteo (Teriparatide) daily injected Recombinant DNA-derived parathyroid hormone or PTH, works by increasing the number of active osteoblasts (bone-building cells), decreasing the natural programmed death of osteoblasts, and recruiting bone-lining cells as osteoblasts, creating bone-building over-activity.
- Protelos (strontium ranelate) is a trace element combined with the synthetic molecule ranelic acid.
- Miacalcin and Fortical are synthetic recombinant DNA nasal spray forms of Calcitonin, first approved by the FDA in 1988.

Origins of Osteoporosis Drugs

Before Dr. Herbert Fleisch discovered that bisphosphonates could be used as an osteoporosis treatment, they were only used as industrial inhibitors of corrosion or sometimes in other industries to prevent scaling through inhibition of calcium carbonate precipitation.

http://press.endocrine.org/doi/abs/10.1210/edrv.19.1.0325

The newest reports about the dangerous side effects of the bisphosphonate drugs are shocking to anyone who does not understand how they work, but utterly unsurprising to those who do.

http://press.endocrine.org/doi/full/10.1210/jc.2005-0057

Most people think of bones as not being a metabolically active tissue because they are used as a hard support structure for the body, but nothing could be further from the truth. Bone is continually being remodeled and turned over to keep it young and flexible, in a healthy person with good bone health. This remodeling process involves old, dried-out, brittle bone constantly being removed from the bone matrix to be resorbed by the body to make room for new, younger, stronger, more flexible bone to be laid down in its place.

Bone cells called *osteoclasts* do the removing of old bone and others called *osteoblasts* do the depositing of new bone. In fact, 5 to 10% of the total bone in the body is replaced each year in this remodeling process. Because bone is so active in rejuvenating itself, it consumes substantial amounts of energy. CoQ-10 can help to support mitochondrial health so that sufficient energy is produced for this process. Bone is even beginning to be recognized as an endocrine organ.

The reason that bone is now considered an endocrine organ is due to osteocalcin acting as a hormone in energy regulation, insulin resistance, and cardiovascular risk.

http://www.ncbi.nlm.nih.gov/pmc/articles/PMC3854658/
http://dx.doi.org/10.1155/2013/197519
http://www.ncbi.nlm.nih.gov/pubmed/21433069

Quality is Much More Important than Quantity When It Comes to Bones

BMD tests such as DXA scans only measure density, which is the thickness or volume of bone. While this gives the doctor something objective to measure, it does <u>not</u> give an accurate representation of bone strength, which has two aspects:

- The first aspect is compression strength, relating to the amount of weight that a bone could hold up before breaking
- But the better indicator of whether or not bones would break is the tensile strength, measuring the flexibility the bone has, or how much the bone could flex before breaking.

Which would you rather have? Thick bones or strong ones?

A bone can be thick, brittle, worn out, dried-up, older, and easy to snap. Or slightly less dense, flexible, younger, and more likely to bend than to break.

Potential Side Effects by Class of Drug

These lists are neither exhaustive nor complete lists of all possible side effects of these drugs, but only a subset of some of the most serious of them.

Bisphosphonates

Osteonecrosis of the jaw and atypical femoral fractures are the most serious of the side effects seen with this class of drugs. Increased risk of kidney failure and atrial fibrillation (muscles of the heart not beating properly in sequence) are possible serious side effects of Reclast. These far overshadow all others, which include the risk of:

- Nausea
- Flatulence
- Generalized pain of the muscles, joints and/or bones
- Heartburn or difficulty swallowing
- Inflammation and ulceration of the esophagus
- Esophageal cancer
- Blood clotting disorders
- Abdominal cramping

- Blurred vision
- Chest pain
- Skin rash
- Flu-like symptoms
- Fever
- Anemia
- Decreased mobility of joints

Evista and Duavee

Evista and Duavee can increase risk of blood clots and stroke, like any other synthetic hormone such as birth control pills. In addition, women have reported hot flashes while taking Evista.

Prolia

Prolia carries a similar risk of osteonecrosis of the jaw as bisphosphonates, but long-term use also has possible effects on the skin and immune system, such as eczema and cellulitis caused by suppression of TRAIL, (TNF-related apoptosis inducing ligand). Patients treated with denosumab have a slightly greater risk of recurrent neoplasms (tumors). Other side effects include low calcium levels, serious skin, lower abdomen, bladder, or ear infections, and inflammation of the inner lining of the heart (endocarditis) caused by an infection.

Forteo

Forteo carries the possible risk of a rare bone cancer called osteosarcoma, caused by an abnormal proliferation of osteoblasts or bone-forming cells, which the drug label states that the rats developed during testing. This is why Forteo is prescribed only for a maximum of two years.

Forteo's other serious side effects include:
- Decrease in blood pressure when you change positions (postural hypotension).
- Increased calcium in your blood. Tell your healthcare provider if you have nausea, vomiting, constipation, low energy, or muscle weakness. These may be signs there is too much calcium in your blood.
- Hair loss, shingles, thyroid problems, muscle and joint aches, constipation, and racing heartbeat.

Protelos

Protelos or Osseor is the brand name of Strontium Ranelate, which has been used in Europe. The newer insert in boxes of Strontium Ranelate has been redesigned and now states "Possible side effects: Common: Blood clots." Common side effects are those that may affect up to 1 in 10 people.

In January 2014, the Risk Assessment Committee of the European Medicines Agency issued a warning to consumers and recommended that strontium should no longer be used to treat osteoporosis in Europe, having identified significant risks, such as heart problems, blood clots, blood vessel blockages, reduced number of blood cells, liver inflammation, seizures, disturbances in consciousness, and serious skin reactions.
http://www.ema.europa.eu/docs/en_GB/document_library /Referrals_document/Protelos_and_Osseor/Recommendati on_provided_by_Pharmacovigilance_Risk_Assessment_Co mmittee/WC500159374.pdf

However, in February 2014, the final recommendations from the Agency's Committee for Medicinal Products for Human Use (CHMP) were to further restrict use, rather than to ban strontium altogether. The European Commission endorsed them, issuing a final legally binding decision valid throughout the European Union.
http://www.ema.europa.eu/ema/index.jsp?curl=pages/medi cines/human/referrals/Protelos_and_Osseor/human_referr al_prac_000025.jsp&mid=WC0b01ac05805c516f

As early as April 2012, Charles T. Price, M.D., Founder of the Institute for Better Bone Health, had previously warned of these concerns in a scientific publication.
http://www.ncbi.nlm.nih.gov/pmc/articles/PMC3330619/

A video is available on the website of the Institute for Better Bone Health as well.
http://www.bonehealthnow.com/cms/QuestionableNutrient sInSupplements_70.aspx

Although strontium ranelate is not approved for use in the United States, commonly used over-the-counter bone health supplement products are available that contain strontium citrate. This form of strontium is especially concerning, given that more of it is taken into the body than a comparable amount of strontium ranelate.

Worse, if you have <u>ever</u> taken strontium in either form, your bone density scan results will not be interpreted accurately, and it may vary according to the equipment used as well.
http://www.ncbi.nlm.nih.gov/pubmed/17543560
http://www.ncbi.nlm.nih.gov/pubmed/10677790
http://www.ncbi.nlm.nih.gov/pubmed/20699129

This is because the strontium atom is a heavier element than calcium, with a larger atomic weight, so it displaces calcium atoms in your bones, inflating the BMD results. As much as 75% of the increase in BMD could be an artifact of strontium.
http://press.endocrine.org/doi/full/10.1210/jcem.87.5.8507
http://www.ncbi.nlm.nih.gov/pubmed/16939400

Unless the radiologist knows that you have taken strontium, your BMD would be overestimated, reflecting a higher result than it should. Not only that, but radiologists are not taught in medical school or residency how to correct for this overestimation, even if you disclose your strontium use.

Scare Tactics Used by Doctors

If you balk at taking the osteoporosis drug that your doctor wants you to take, you will likely encounter the scare tactics that most doctors will resort to in order to get you to comply. These are just a few of the remarks that you can expect to hear:

- *"If you don't take Evista, sooner or later, you'll fall and break a hip, maybe end up in a wheel chair or eventually die."*
- *"Your DXA scan shows that you have osteopenia. You need to take Actonel to stop the bone loss."*
- *"If you don't take Boniva, your bones are going to get so weakened that you'll get fractures just climbing up stairs or turning over in bed."*
- *"If you don't take Reclast, you'll become ugly and hunch-backed from your weakened bones."*
- *"Look, the Prolia will only need to be injected twice a year. Why not be safe instead of sorry?"*

SSRI Antidepressants

SSRIs include citalopram (Celexa), dapoxetine (Priligy), escitalopram (Lexapro), fluoxetine (Prozac), fluvoxamine (Luvox), paroxetine (Paxil), sertraline (Zoloft) and the like. In the most recent observational cross-sectional study on this subject published in the journal *Osteoporosis International*, the link between Selective Serotonin Reuptake Inhibitors (SSRIs) and bone health decline continues to be found. In fact, a November 2014 study found that the rate of failure of dental implants, which depends on osseointegration, shown to be influenced by bone metabolism, was over twice as much in SSRI users, 4.6% for SSRI nonusers and 10.6% for SSRI users.
http://www.ncbi.nlm.nih.gov/pubmed/25187118
http://www.ncbi.nlm.nih.gov/pubmed/25186831
http://dx.doi.org/10.1155/2012/323061

PPIs for GERD (Acid Reflux)

Acid reflux medications such as the Proton Pump Inhibitors (PPIs) Nexium, Prilosec, and Prevacid also increase fracture risks. In fact, after two years, risk is increased by 41% and almost 60% after four years of taking these medicines. One study estimated that for every ten women taking PPIs for five years, there would be one extra non-spine fracture.
http://www.ncbi.nlm.nih.gov/pubmed/21555754
http://www.ncbi.nlm.nih.gov/pubmed/21185417
http://www.ncbi.nlm.nih.gov/pubmed/18813868
http://www.ncbi.nlm.nih.gov/pubmed/20458083
http://www.ncbi.nlm.nih.gov/pubmed/22392829
http://www.ncbi.nlm.nih.gov/pubmed/17190895
http://www.ncbi.nlm.nih.gov/pmc/articles/PMC2596870

PPI use reduced the fractional absorption of calcium from 9.1% to 3.5% in one 2005 study, so that decrease in absorption could be the mechanism by which the risk is increased.
http://www.ncbi.nlm.nih.gov/pubmed/15989913

Alternatives to PPIs include H2 receptor blockers such as Zantac. The risk of fractures seems lower with these types of acid reducers, possibly owing to less acid being blocked with these older medications. However, even with these, one study in men did show increased risk for fracture.

http://www.ncbi.nlm.nih.gov/pubmed/9143208

Depo-Provera Birth Control Injection

The FDA has issued a black box warning about the negative effects of this medication on bone health. Despite this, an American College of Obstetricians and Gynecologists Committee on Gynecologic Practice published opinion still recommended to continue to prescribe it, even for adolescents for whom the future bone health risk is unknown. Not even one doctor's name is signed to that opinion. I wouldn't either, considering that the inevitable lawsuits have already begun.
http://www.ncbi.nlm.nih.gov/pubmed/18929733
http://www.ncbi.nlm.nih.gov/pubmed/24848921
http://www.ncbi.nlm.nih.gov/pubmed/24640465

Corticosteroids Such as Cortisone

Here's another acronym for you: GIO, or glucocorticoid-induced osteoporosis. Steroid therapy such as cortisone, methylprednisolone dexamethasone, prednisone, and hydrocortisone increase your risk. More than three months of cortisone therapy such as those used for asthma, Crohn's disease, or arthritis treatment increases total risk of fractures without regard to bone density. One study predicted a 62% increased fracture risk for every 10 mg rise in dosage.
http://www.ncbi.nlm.nih.gov/pubmed/20218181
http://www.ncbi.nlm.nih.gov/pubmed/10841167
http://www.ncbi.nlm.nih.gov/pubmed/12952387

In 1996, the American College of Rheumatology Task Force on Osteoporosis Guidelines estimated that 20% of all the cases of osteoporosis at the time could be attributed to corticosteroid use. That was 4 million cases!
http://www.ncbi.nlm.nih.gov/pubmed/8912500

Something to think about: Your body produces cortisol in response to worry and stress. Cortisol has the same effect on bones as the steroids do. Interestingly, there is even a scripture that predicted this. *A merry heart is like a medicine, but a broken spirit drieth the bones.* (Proverbs 17:22)

If we decide to enjoy life no matter what, to find our joy in everyday pleasures, it will show up in our very bones!

Broad Spectrum Antibiotics

Because Vitamin K2 is synthesized in the gut through microbial sources, taking antibiotics can reduce your levels 75% by changing the vitamin K2 producing gut microbiome.
http://www.ncbi.nlm.nih.gov/pubmed/7752839

Diabetes Medications and Insulin

Actos and Avandia can increase fracture risk by 57% after only one year of use, according to the *Journal of Clinical Endocrinology & Metabolism*. The increased risk is 72% in those 65 or older. Insulin-dependent diabetics are also at increased risk.
http://dx.doi.org/10.1210/jc.2009-1385
http://www.ncbi.nlm.nih.gov/pubmed/11423502

Other Medications and Bone Problems

Several other medications also can interact with bone formation or strength: bipolar medications such as lithium, epilepsy medications such as phenobarbital, OTC antacids that contain aluminum, and immunosuppressants. And here's another one I'll bet you haven't heard about. Acetaminophen (Tylenol, Excedrin) use is linked to increased risk of fractures.
http://www.ncbi.nlm.nih.gov/pubmed/21396491
http://www.ncbi.nlm.nih.gov/pubmed/21710339

Medical Conditions Causing Bone Problems

A 15-year study published in 2014 showed that over half of celiac patients had bone health problems.
http://www.ncbi.nlm.nih.gov/pubmed/25404189

Another 2014 study measured BMD on diagnosis of celiac and again after one year of a gluten-free diet, with significant improvement after avoiding gluten.
http://www.ncbi.nlm.nih.gov/pubmed/25379519

Cushing's disease, inflammatory bowel disease such as Crohn's and ulcerative colitis, rheumatoid arthritis, insulin-dependent diabetes, MS, lactose intolerance, leukemia, COPD, gastric bypass, lymphoma, stroke, anorexia, and primary biliary cirrhosis also increase risk.

Part 3

Better Ways to Improve Bone Health

"It's not what happens to you; it's what you do about it that makes the difference." **W. Mitchell**

Wouldn't it be wonderful to know that you were not only reducing your age-related bone loss and the associated risk of fractures, but also restoring your bone mineral density to healthy levels? Four actions can make that a reality for you:

1. Take Vitamin K2 (always with Vitamin D3 [or 15-20 minutes of sunshine] and Vitamin A), especially if taking calcium supplements.

2. Reduce or eliminate the drugs you are taking that can endanger your bone health, such as SSRIs, certain popular blood thinners such as warfarin (Coumadin), and even GERD (acid reflux) medications.

3. Get adequate sleep, at least 6 hours, preferably 8 hours, which is a real problem for many today.

4. Get adequate sun (15-20 minutes a day) **without sunscreen** or if that is impossible, take Vitamin D in the optimal form, D3, but only with Vitamin A also.

The most important are Vitamins K2, D3, and A.

Because they are all fat-soluble, taking Vitamins D3, A, and K2 with adequate fat is important for optimal absorption. Vitamin D3 requires Vitamin K2 for proper synthesis. Vitamins D3 and A prevent toxicity for each other, so always take all three for optimal results.
http://www.ncbi.nlm.nih.gov/pubmed/17145139

Bone Supplements

Supple-ment	Preferred Type	Suggested Daily Amount
Vitamin K2	MK-4	15 mg in 3 doses of 5 mg each if no bone loss unless taking warfarin (or other Vitamin K-affecting blood thinners). (See section on Vitamin K2 and Warfarin.)
		45 mg (45,000 mcg) in three doses of 15 mg each if bone loss has begun unless taking warfarin (or other Vitamin K-affecting blood thinners).
	MK-7	45-90 mcg unless taking warfarin (or other Vitamin K-affecting blood thinners). Cees Vermeer recommends a range up to 185 mcg.
Vitamin D3	D3 only	3,000-5,000 IU
Vitamin A	Palmitate	5,000 IU
Calcium	Ca aspartate Ca orotate Ca citrate malate Ca gluconate Ca glycinate Ca lactate Ca malate	1,200 mg elemental calcium from an organic or chelated source
Magnesium	Mg citrate Mg gluconate Mg aspartate Mg glycinate Mg malate Mg taurate	100-200 mg 3 times daily
Co-Enzyme Q-10	Ubiquinol	50 mg (more potent form)
	Ubiquinone Soft gelatin capsule (NOT tablet or powder form)	200 mg
Potassium	Potassium Citrate	2-4 grams, preferably from diet rather than supplements.

Supple-ment	Preferred Type	Suggested Daily Amount
Nettle (Urtica dioica)	Nettle root extract capsules	140 mg
Copper		2 mg
Boron		3 mg unless kidney disease is present
Zinc		15 mg daily

Vitamin K2

Usually, when people think of Vitamin K dietary sources, they think of green leafy vegetables and unhydrogenated vegetable oils, but that form is Vitamin K1, phylloquinone, not the form that has the best effects on bone, which is Vitamin K2, menaquinone. Two different forms of Vitamin K2 are available, menaquinone-4 (MK-4) (found in meats and eggs) and menaquinone-7 (MK-7) (found in cheese and other dairy products, sauerkraut, and natto).
http://dx.doi.org/10.1080/13590849961717

A December 2014 meta-analysis supports K2's role in reversing osteoporosis in postmenopausal women.
http://www.ncbi.nlm.nih.gov/pubmed/25516361

MK-4 Versus MK-7: Which One is Better?

The controversy about this rages on. Cees Vermeer is a respected medical researcher who does prefer MK-7. Yet, I wonder how much the recent development of less expensive commercial MK-7 production plays into this. And with natto (the highest MK-7 food source) so easily available in Japan, I have to wonder why the Japanese researchers would use MK-4 instead in their clinical studies and in the government approved treatments? That is baffling to me unless they know something that I did not find in the medical literature supporting superiority of MK-4. Personally, I am hedging my bets and obtaining half my K2 from each, so no matter which is better, I am getting it.

This chart compares the two Vitamin K-2 forms.

MK-4 and MK-7 Comparison Chart		
Quality	MK-4	MK-7
Can be measured in the blood?	No	Yes
How long it remains in body?	Half is gone in 3-4 hours	Half is gone in 3.5 days
Contained in human breast milk and the brain?	Yes	No
Produced in the body?	Yes	No
Activates transcription of (Upregulates) osteoblastic genes?	Yes, GDF15 and STC2, involved in bone and cartilage formation	Yes, TnC (influences osteoblast adhesion and differentiation) and BMP2 (involved in bone and cartilage formation)

MK-4 activates transcription of two genes in osteoblast cells, GDF15 and STC2, which are involved in bone and cartilage formation. MK-7 did not activate transcription of those genes.
http://www.ncbi.nlm.nih.gov/pubmed/17909264
http://jme.endocrinology-journals.org/content/39/4/239.full.pdf

MK-7 does seem to upregulate other genes in osteoblast cells, including TnC and BMP2. Within bone, TnC (tenascin C) influences osteoblast adhesion and differentiation. BMP2 (bone morphogenetic protein) induces bone and cartilage formation.
http://www.ncbi.nlm.nih.gov/pubmed/17203202

In order for osteocalcin to attach itself to bone to create new bone tissue, it must be carboxylated by Vitamin K2. In order for Matrix Gla-Protein (MGP) to sweep calcium out of soft tissues, it must be carboxylated by Vitamin K2. This is the cardiovascular protective effect of K2. Population-based studies have shown that MK-7 and other long-chain menaquinones had a more potent cardioprotective effect than the shorter chain MK-4. This was concluded because smaller doses of it were required to counteract warfarin-induced calcification.

MK-4 and Mk-7 have different dosages that are effective to carboxylate osteocalcin. In one study, MK-4 at 500 mcg did not do the job, and a dosage of 1500 mcg was required to show the desired effects of osteocalcin carboxylation. For MK-7, it only took 45 to 90 mcg to be effective.

Takeuchi A, Masuda Y, Kimura M, Marushima R, Matsuoka R, et al. (2005) Minimal effective dose of vitamin K2 (menaquinone-4) on serum osteocalcin concentration in Japanese subjects and safety evaluation of vitamin K2 supplemented in calcium tablet. J Jpn Soc Clin Nutr 26: 254-260.
http://www.ncbi.nlm.nih.gov/pubmed/19450370
http://www.ncbi.nlm.nih.gov/pubmed/21736837
http://www.ncbi.nlm.nih.gov/pubmed/21628633
http://www.ncbi.nlm.nih.gov/pubmed/22819559

The brain preferentially accumulates MK-4, but not MK-7. Vitamin K1 is converted by the human body into small amounts of MK-4, but not MK-7. Human breast milk contains MK-4, but not MK-7. After supplementation, MK-7 can be measured in the blood serum, but MK-4 cannot.
http://www.ncbi.nlm.nih.gov/pubmed/12064330
http://www.ncbi.nlm.nih.gov/pubmed/23140417

Some researchers concluded that MK-7 is a better supplier of MK-4 to tissues outside the liver because when the same dose of MK-7 and MK-4 is given, only those given MK-7 have elevated MK-4 found in extrahepatic tissues. However, it takes more MK-4 to be effective, as evidenced by the preceding carboxylation studies. It could be that MK-4 is more easily taken into cells and used (bioavailable) and therefore is not still detected in tissues after a short time.
http://www.ncbi.nlm.nih.gov/pubmed/1297781
http://www.ncbi.nlm.nih.gov/pubmed/20953171
http://www.ncbi.nlm.nih.gov/pmc/articles/PMC3502319/

MK-4 K2 Sources

If you have no bone loss yet, the lower dose of MK-4 can be taken in three doses per day of 5 mg each. This dose is found in these capsules:

http://www.amazon.com/dp/B003B3P4I6
Carlson Labs MK-4, 5 mg capsules, 180 count
Two months' doses $34

If you have bone loss already, the larger 45 mg daily dose of MK-4 can be difficult to find. I first took this liquid version:
http://www.amazon.com/dp/B000FGWDTK
Thorne Research Liquid MK-4 K2, 75 doses of 15 mg
Almost one month's doses $65

This product, however, is <u>about half the price</u>:
http://www.amazon.com/dp/B00GZVM092
Relentless Improvement MK-4 K2, 90 count, 15 mg capsules
One month's doses $33

If Amazon is out of stock, it is available with $3.95 shipping:
https://supplements.relentlessimprovement.com/vitamin-k2-mk4-menatetrenone-p285.aspx

And if both are out, this one is almost as cost-effective:
http://www.amazon.com/dp/B0057ZGWDW
Complementary Prescriptions Ultra K2, 90 count, 15 mg capsules One month's doses $38

MK-7 K2 Sources

http://www.amazon.com/dp/B002N1MW3W
Doctor's Best 45 mcg, 60 count, Two month's doses $9

http://www.amazon.com/dp/B001KSNDSM
Life Extension, 45 mcg, 90 count, Three month's doses $13

http://www.amazon.com/dp/B000SPF03O
Jarrow, 90 mcg, 60 count, Two month's higher doses $17

Vitamin K2 and Warfarin

Vitamin K can interfere with the anticoagulant action of coumarin derivatives such as the Vitamin K antagonist warfarin, but lower doses appear to be safe if INR is monitored by a health provider. Schurgers et al. recommend an upper safety limit of 50 mcg/d for MK-7 for patients on warfarin treatment. This amount is the same as in 3.5 ounces of cheese, which research indicates would affect INR by .2.

However, as mentioned earlier, switching to an anticoagulant that is not a Vitamin K antagonist would be simpler.
http://www.ncbi.nlm.nih.gov/pubmed/23530987

Vitamin D3

The commercial availability of 25(OH)D tests to determine Vitamin D3 levels in the body has brought the need for this nutrient front and center. According to Dr. Robert Heaney, one of the major researchers and pioneers in this field, 99% of what we have learned about Vitamin D was in the last 10 years, due to the fact that we finally had an available assay to measure it.
http://www.ncbi.nlm.nih.gov/pubmed/17218096

Aim for reaching optimal levels of D3, in the range of 60-80 ng/mL or 150 to 200 nmol/l. (1 nmol/L = 0.4 ng/mL)
http://www.ncbi.nlm.nih.gov/pubmed/15776217/

A meta-analysis of controlled trials demonstrated no benefit in reducing risk of osteoporotic fracture unless serum 25(OH)D reached at least 75 nmol/L (30 ng/mL).
http://www.ncbi.nlm.nih.gov/pubmed/19307517

Using a loading dose of D3 when deficiency exists, to quickly get levels to optimal, is beginning to be used, especially in elderly populations and the obese, who do not absorb as well.
http://www.ncbi.nlm.nih.gov/pubmed/22426953
http://www.ncbi.nlm.nih.gov/pubmed/18991184
http://www.ncbi.nlm.nih.gov/pubmed/19539796
http://www.ncbi.nlm.nih.gov/pubmed/20565345
http://www.ncbi.nlm.nih.gov/pubmed/15992330

To get a higher dose, such as 50,000 IU, I found a few sources for non-prescription D3:
http://www.amazon.com/dp/B00LXNU684
http://www.amazon.com/dp/B003I90G36
http://www.amazon.com/dp/B008KZD6EO
http://www.amazon.com/dp/B002V0LHI6

The type of vitamin D that you get from sun exposure, Vitamin D3 (Cholecalciferol), is the bioactive kind of Vitamin D. However, few doctors know this and even if they are aware enough to test you for Vitamin D levels, they are likely to prescribe pharmaceutical doses of Vitamin D2. You want D3.

Vitamin D3 is a vitamin that acts as a hormone, with the following benefits:
- Reduces risk of breaking a bone in any part of the body by 33%.
- Reduces risk of a breaking a hip by 69%.

Vitamin D3 helps calcium to be absorbed as well as being important for immunity and having antibiotic-like actions. Moreover, it has been found to be biochemically safe in high doses, even up to 40,000 IU daily for brief periods or 10,000 IU daily for a year.
http://www.ncbi.nlm.nih.gov/pubmed/24425848
http://www.ncbi.nlm.nih.gov/pubmed/23413544
http://dx.doi.org/10.1097/01.NT.0000380924.55670.b1

To make Vitamin D, your body needs cholesterol, because the precursor molecule 7-dehydrocholesterol is in the same metabolic pathway as cholesterol. The higher your cholesterol level, the more vitamin D your body can make. Since most people are being told to lower their cholesterol levels through use of statin drugs, this will affect the body's ability to manufacture Vitamin D3. I'll discuss the cholesterol and statins lie in a later book in this series, one on the subject of heart disease.

Add to this the fact that many are taking other drugs such as corticosteroids that deplete Vitamin D3. Elevated cortisol caused by stress has the same effect. Or eating a low-fat diet that makes it difficult to absorb fat-soluble vitamins such as D3, A, and K2, as they require the presence of dietary lipids and bile to help the vitamins get absorbed in the intestines.

Sun exposure is something that many avoid because of fear of skin cancer, but if 15-20 minutes of sun exposure without sunscreen was so dangerous, would scientists have used it in these clinical trials?
http://www.ncbi.nlm.nih.gov/pubmed/21682695
http://www.ncbi.nlm.nih.gov/pubmed/19959915
http://www.ncbi.nlm.nih.gov/pubmed/16007329
http://www.ncbi.nlm.nih.gov/pubmed/12913194

And remember all that calcium you've been taking and trying to include in your diet for years now? If you are Vitamin D deficient, you only absorbed 10-15% of it and most was wasted. If you have adequate Vitamin D, you absorb 30-40%.
http://www.ncbi.nlm.nih.gov/pubmed/12672710

Not only that, but Vitamin D protects against Vitamin A toxicity. They need to be taken together in an A to D ratio somewhere between 4 to 1 and 8 to 1, as in the 5 to 1 ratio found in Blue Ice High Vitamin Cod Liver Oil.
http://www.amazon.com/dp/B002LZYPS0

Food sources for Vitamin D are shellfish, oily fish, lard from pastured pigs, and egg yolks from pastured chickens.

Vitamin A

According to a 2008 study published in the Journal of Nutrition, Vitamin A also protects against Vitamin D toxicity. It does this by curbing excess production of MGP that is triggered by Vitamin D intake. It also prevents the kidney stones that can result from Vitamin D supplementation without adding Vitamin A. Excessive MGP increases need for Vitamin K2 to carboxylate it to prevent calcification of soft tissues.
http://www.ncbi.nlm.nih.gov/pubmed/19022954
http://www.amazon.com/dp/B00OVZ1D6Y

Food sources of Vitamin A include egg yolks, organ meats such as liver, sweet potatoes, carrots, collard greens, kale, butternut squash, romaine lettuce, cantaloupe, and apricots.

Magnesium

Sufficient magnesium is important to maintain the balance between it and calcium because taking high levels of Vitamin D3 will allow your body to absorb significantly more calcium. These two minerals counterbalance each other in many cellular functions.
http://www.ncbi.nlm.nih.gov/pubmed/11398593

Symptoms of magnesium deficiency include elevated blood pressure, transient ischemic attacks (TIA), heart arrhythmia, migraines and tension headaches, muscle weakness, leg cramps, and restless legs.

Food sources for magnesium are whole seeds such as legumes, nuts, whole grains, seafood, and leafy green vegetables. People with heart or kidney problems should only take supplements with medical supervision.
http://www.amazon.com/dp/B000BD0RT0

Copper

In order for calcium to adhere properly to the collagen matrix of bone, adequate copper must be present, which was first discovered by Robert O. Becker in the mid-1980's.
http://www.ncbi.nlm.nih.gov/pubmed/12133199
http://www.ncbi.nlm.nih.gov/pubmed/8409100

Cattle with adequate levels of calcium still developed rickets and soft bones if they did not have sufficient copper in the diet.
http://www.ncbi.nlm.nih.gov/pmc/articles/PMC1578155/pdf/califmed00099-0135a.pdf

Best food sources of copper are lobster and oysters. Seeds, nuts, mushrooms, and dried beans are less potent sources.
http://www.amazon.com/dp/B00014D8UE

CoQ10

CoQ10 is one of the most powerful antioxidants, present in almost all cell membranes and responsible for energy production in the form of ATP (adenosine triphosphate) for your mitochondria, the powerhouse of the cells. Without this essential energy, bone-building is less effective.
http://www.amazon.com/dp/B00014I4XMS

Boron

Boron tends to normalize magnesium and calcium levels to influence bone metabolism and is also known for normalizing hormone levels in older adults. The tolerable UL (upper limit) is 20 mg. Boron can be a problem if you have kidney disease or your kidneys are not working well, because your kidneys need to work hard to eliminate boron from your body. Best food sources are avocados, cherries and grapes, scallops, mussels, clams, almonds, peanuts, and hazelnuts.

http://www.ncbi.nlm.nih.gov/pubmed/2222801
http://www.ncbi.nlm.nih.gov/pmc/articles/PMC1566639
http://www.amazon.com/dp/B00093D2NU

Zinc

Zinc is a crucial mineral for normal collagen synthesis and mineralization of bone. If you take amiloride, prednisone, cyclosporine, or any other medicine that suppresses your immune system (immunosuppressant), you shouldn't take zinc supplements without talking to your physician first.
http://www.ncbi.nlm.nih.gov/pmc/articles/PMC3995959

Oysters, grass-fed beef, wheat germ, and whole grains contain zinc.
http://www.ncbi.nlm.nih.gov/pubmed/24602492
http://www.amazon.com/dp/B000I4DQM2

Potassium

Potassium citrate (NOT potassium chloride) at a dosage of 60 mEq, which is 6480 mg, was shown to decrease fractures in a 2012 study, but that is a pharmacological dosage. Over the counter potassium citrate comes in 99 mg pills, so that would be quite difficult (and possibly problematic) to obtain and safely ingest, absent a prescription and medical monitoring.

Since potassium balance is critical, too much potassium can cause your heart to stop. But, in a healthy body, your kidneys should regulate your levels and excrete any extra you might have in the urine. If your potassium is too low, it can cause headache, tiredness, muscle weakness, and mental confusion.

I suggest eating more fresh fruits and vegetables to raise potassium citrate levels naturally. Best food sources include bananas, cantaloupes, cabbage, oranges, spinach, and celery.

People with kidney problems or diabetes, as well as those taking NSAIDs, heparin, ACE inhibitors, or potassium-sparing diuretics, should only take potassium supplements with medical supervision.
http://www.ncbi.nlm.nih.gov/pubmed/23162100
http://www.ncbi.nlm.nih.gov/pubmed/15817873

Nettle

Nettle is important because it contains a compound that can bind with a protein called SHBG to lower its levels in your body. Why would you want to do that? In most people, only 2% of the testosterone in the body is available because the rest is bound to SHBG. Aging increases levels of SHBG, which then decreases free testosterone in the body by binding to it, making it unavailable to bind to androgen receptors. The estrogen-mimics in the environment also cause SHBG levels to rise.

Testosterone supports bone-building (not to mention libido). The root extract is most potent form, containing at least 65% nettle.
http://www.amazon.com/dp/B000I48PTG

Calcium

Organic/chelated is the preferred form of calcium.
http://www.amazon.com/dp/B00DECMOGO
http://www.amazon.com/dp/B00IOEOPF0

Food sources for calcium include dairy products, canned sardines or salmon with bones, beans, broccoli, collard greens, kale, mustard greens, butternut squash, and sweet potatoes. I recommend full fat dairy, not low-fat, and of course, hormone-free.

Harvard School of Public Health reported that when we were eating 45% fat, 13% were obese and less than 1% had diabetes. Reducing the fat to 33% resulted in 34% obesity rates and 8% diabetes incidence. Do you think that's a coincidence? I don't.
http://tinyurl.com/PerCentFat

Adequate Protein

All of the focus on calcium for the last decade has seemed to cause people to forget that bone is 50 percent protein by volume. Bone is only about 20 percent calcium by weight.
http://blogs.creighton.edu/heaney/2014/07/25/the-paradox-of-osteoporosis-irreversibility-2/

Protein is essential for the bone matrix formation before bone minerals are laid down on that framework. It also makes it easier for your bones to absorb calcium.
http://ajcn.nutrition.org/content/87/5/1567S.full
http://jn.nutrition.org/content/133/3/855S.full
http://press.endocrine.org/doi/full/10.1210/jc.2003-031466

No matter how much calcium or other nutrients you take, if the bone matrix is not healthy, you won't build healthy bones. And that requires collagen, which requires animal protein sources to be produced reliably. If you leave adequate protein out of your diet, reversing bone loss can be impossible.

Be sure to opt for the healthiest animal protein sources you can afford, such as beef that is grass-fed, hormone-free, antibiotic-free, free-range chickens, cage-free eggs, and pastured dairy.

Many studies show that people who eat the most protein have the slowest bone loss over time and that people who eat the most protein have the lowest fracture rate over time.
http://www.ncbi.nlm.nih.gov/pubmed/11127216
http://www.ncbi.nlm.nih.gov/pmc/articles/PMC3179277/
http://www.ncbi.nlm.nih.gov/pubmed/22127335

Weight-Bearing Exercise

A high-intensity interval training routine such as Metabolic Aftershock could be the most efficient way to accomplish the necessary weight-bearing exercise without the burdensome time commitment of traditional cardio, jogging, or running.
http://www.thisclickrocks.com/ma

I know what some of you might be thinking, "Come on, I am not in good enough shape to do anything high-intensity, even for 15 minutes 3 times a week."

However, you would be surprised at just how little effort is really required to keep your bones strong with exercise. Back extensor muscle strength is important for healthy bones. In a randomized controlled trial study first conducted from 1987 to 1989 at the Mayo Clinic, 50 postmenopausal women were divided into two groups, 27 that exercised and 23 that did not.

The exercise group did a simple back-strengthening exercise in which they laid down on their stomachs and lifted their upper bodies off the ground 10 times without using their arms, while wearing backpacks with progressively heavier weights in them as time went on, up to 50 pounds at max.

They did this for two years, five times a week. The first results were not impressive at all, with no significant differences in the two groups in terms of bone mineral density, but the exercising group increased back extensor strength by 70% compared to the control group, which only increased by 32%. http://www.ncbi.nlm.nih.gov/pubmed/2671517

"So what?" you might ask. Well, here's the reason you want to know about this study. Mayo Clinic did a follow-up study several years later that showed significant differences between the two groups in terms of spinal compression fracture rates. Eight years after they stopped the exercise program, the exercise group's fracture rates were much lower. In fact, the relative risk for compression fracture was 2.7 times greater in the control group than in the group that had exercised *8 years earlier*. And ten years later, the difference in back strength was still significant. Not only that, but also the exercising group's bone density was significantly greater, although it had not been significantly better than the controls at the end of the original study. http://www.ncbi.nlm.nih.gov/pubmed/12052450

This simple, fast, exercise routine had long-lasting effects for bone health even years after discontinuation. So if you think that you don't have time to exercise for your bones, you do, if you do this super-quick and easy routine. It really doesn't have to be time-consuming or complicated to make a difference.

Whole Body Vibration

A new technology is another alternative to (for those who are restricted in movement) or addition to exercise: whole body vibration. This technology is a way to deliver mechanical challenges to the weight-bearing skeleton without requiring movement. When I first researched this years ago, the only machine to do this was called Power Plate, and it cost thousands of dollars, so this substantial investment put it out of reach of many.

Luckily, lower cost versions are available now.
http://www.amazon.com/dp/B001FQ8SMU
http://www.amazon.com/dp/B000Y0AMCM

Russian cosmonauts have used this technology to prevent bone loss induced by low-gravity environments in space. The low intensity vibration needs to be not more than 0.3g at 30Hz, not to exceed 30 minutes a day. A 24-week study of postmenopausal women demonstrated strength increases similar to that of weighted exercises. Muscle speed and responsiveness increased <u>more</u> than with weighted workouts.
http://www.ncbi.nlm.nih.gov/pubmed/15040822
http://www.ncbi.nlm.nih.gov/pubmed/19439517
http://www.ncbi.nlm.nih.gov/pubmed/17595419
http://www.ncbi.nlm.nih.gov/pmc/articles/PMC3586310
http://www.ncbi.nlm.nih.gov/pubmed/25317067

Sleep

In women older than 45, a 2011 study showed correlation between lower BMD and 6 hours or less of sleep per night.
http://dx.doi.org/10.1016/j.bone.2011.08.008

In addition to this finding, a rat study done in 2012 found bone formation and marrow abnormalities had resulted from inadequate sleep.
http://dx.doi.org/10.1258/ebm.2012.012043

A 2014 study found that sleep disorders can also play a part in bone health. http://dx.doi.org/10.1016/j.sleep.2014.07.005

The sleep disorder called OSA (Obstructive Sleep Apnea) is associated with 2.74 times the risk of osteoporosis than for patients without it, in another 2014 study.
http://dx.doi.org/10.1210/jc.2014-1718

What to Avoid

Avoid fluoride at the dentist and in toothpastes, as well as in the water supply. Avoid aluminum in deodorants and in cookware.

http://www.ncbi.nlm.nih.gov/pubmed/2018020
http://www.ncbi.nlm.nih.gov/pubmed/24777741
http://www.ncbi.nlm.nih.gov/pubmed/2018020
http://www.hindawi.com/journals/isrn/2013/517601/
http://www.ncbi.nlm.nih.gov/pubmed/11464651

A Breakthrough Anti-Aging Supplement

I cannot end this book without letting you know that a fairly new supplement, PQQ (pyrroloquinoline quinone), has been discovered – one that can help your body to produce new mitochondria. It has long been thought that increasing numbers of mitochondria in the body was impossible. Mitochondria are vitally important to your health in so many ways, because they are the cell's energy producer.

Although Vitamin K2 is a great anti-aging supplement in addition to its bone-building advantages, PQQ can do something for preventing effects of aging that no other supplement can do, because no other has been proven to stimulate mitochondrial biogenesis. Since this information is so recent, very few even know about it yet, but now you do. A very few sources of PQQ are available now:

PQQ alone
http://www.amazon.com/dp/B00C1E7SHQ

PQQ with CoQ10
http://www.amazon.com/dp/B006XJCHLW
http://www.amazon.com/dp/B006JSR00U

My wish for all of you is that you are healthy forever, because you have worked hard for the healthy body of your dreams. More and healthier mitochondria will help to get you there.

You Deserve to Be Healthy

That was a wild ride, wasn't it? I realize that much of what you read in this book, like most of my books, is not common knowledge. Discovering that what your doctor recommended to you might not be the best advice is eye-opening, possibly even inconceivable to many of you before reading this book. But keep in mind that I have backed it all up with valid research, randomized controlled trials, clinical studies, and other credible sources for my facts.

People are so health-conscious these days, and I am glad to see it. Unfortunately, however, I'm also appalled that we have been given such inferior information from our trusted medical advisors and mainstream medicine upon which to base that health quest.

It breaks my heart to see you doing your best to be healthy, but doing all the things that I know are not going to get you there. This book and the rest of the books in this series on other health challenges are my contribution to the world to make it easier to get the results we all want for the best health possible.

You deserve to enjoy the healthy life that you have worked so hard to obtain. I want to help you to have the healthy life you earned. If I have helped to make that possible for you through this book, then my prayer has been answered.

Also by Harmony Clearwater Grace

HCG Diet Made Simple
Your Step-By-Step Guide Beyond Pounds and Inches
5th Edition
http://www.amazon.com/dp/098226674X

The HCG Diet Book of Secrets
Stabilizing After HCG and Staying Slim Forever
http://www.amazon.com/dp/0982266731

Paleo on the Cheap
Saving Time and Money While Saving Your Health
http://www.amazon.com/dp/B00A1X2GQM

Thank you so much for reading my book. I hope you really liked it.

As you probably know, many people look at book reviews before they decide to purchase.

If you liked this book, could you please take a minute to leave a review with your feedback?

You can do that right here: http://thisclickrocks.com/Lies1

60 seconds is all I'm asking for, and it would mean the world to me.

Thank you so much,
Harmony